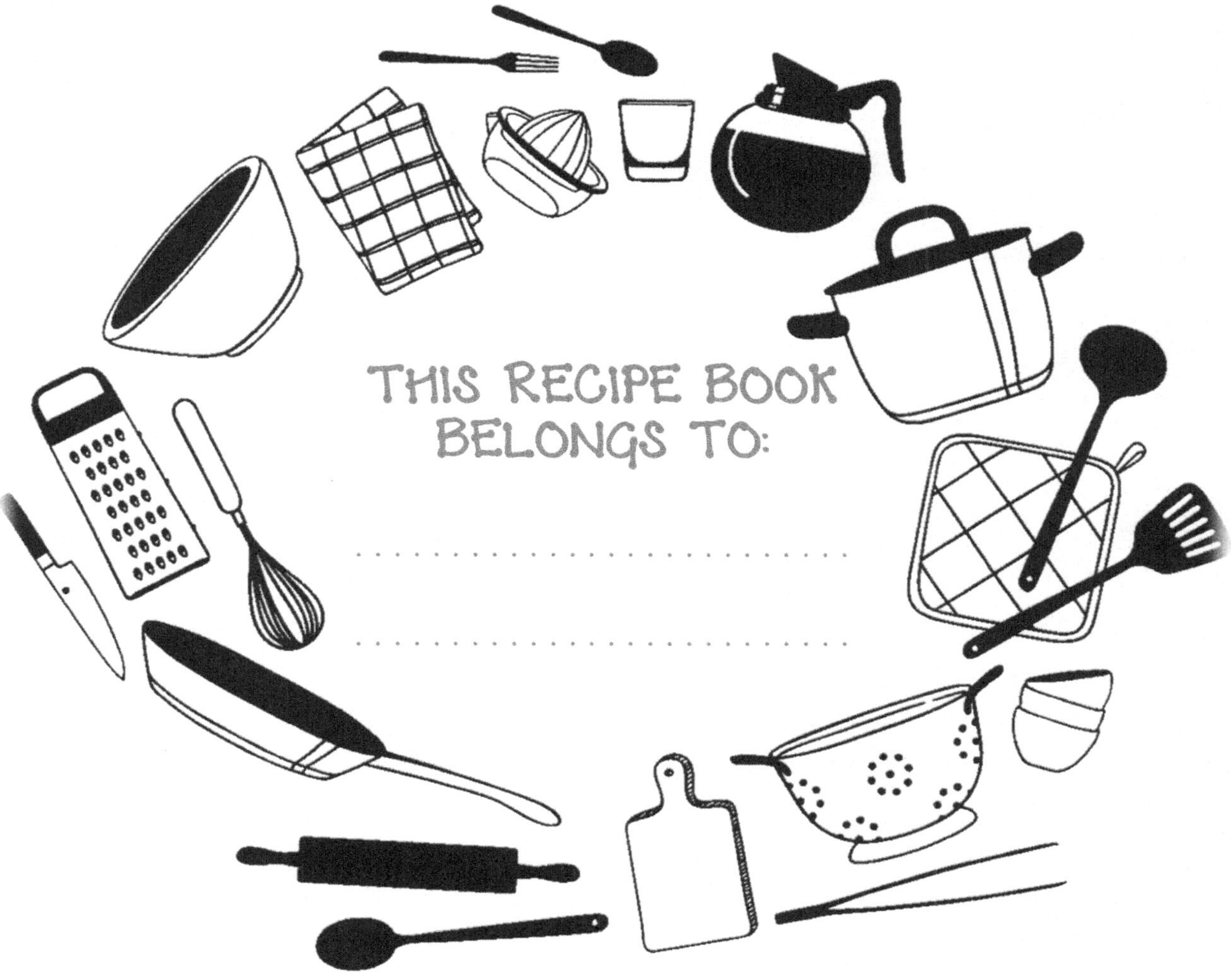

THIS RECIPE BOOK BELONGS TO:

....

....

Copyright © 2019 Billionaire's Blank Cookbooks

Copyright © 2019 Motivational Affirmation Journals

All rights reserved

RECIPE FINDER

Recipe name	Page #	Recipe name	Page #

RECIPE FINDER

Recipe name	Page #	Recipe name	Page #

RECIPE FINDER

Recipe name	Page #	Recipe name	Page #

RECIPE:

Servings   Prep Time   Cook Time

Ingredients   Directions

📓 NOTES

RECIPE:

Servings | Prep Time | Cook Time

Ingredients | Directions

NOTES

RECIPE:

Servings   Prep Time   Cook Time

Ingredients | Directions

NOTES

RECIPE:

Servings Prep Time Cook Time

Ingredients   Directions

NOTES

RECIPE:

Servings | Prep Time | Cook Time

Ingredients

Directions

NOTES

RECIPE:

Servings | Prep Time | Cook Time

Ingredients | Directions

NOTES

RECIPE:

Servings | Prep Time | Cook Time

Ingredients

Directions

NOTES

RECIPE:

Servings | Prep Time | Cook Time

Ingredients | Directions

NOTES

RECIPE:

Servings　　　　　Prep Time　　　　　Cook Time

Ingredients　　Directions

NOTES

RECIPE:

Servings　　　　　Prep Time　　　　　Cook Time

Ingredients　　Directions

NOTES

RECIPE:

Servings Prep Time Cook Time

Ingredients **Directions**

NOTES

RECIPE:

Servings　　　　　　　　Prep Time　　　　　　　　Cook Time

Ingredients　　Directions

NOTES

RECIPE:

Servings Prep Time Cook Time

Ingredients   Directions

NOTES

RECIPE:

Servings Prep Time Cook Time

Ingredients Directions

NOTES

RECIPE:

Servings　　　　　　Prep Time　　　　　　Cook Time

Ingredients　　**Directions**

NOTES

RECIPE:

Servings　　　　　　　Prep Time　　　　　　　Cook Time

Ingredients　　Directions

NOTES

RECIPE:

Servings   Prep Time   Cook Time

Ingredients   Directions

NOTES

RECIPE:

Servings Prep Time Cook Time

Ingredients Directions

NOTES

RECIPE:

Servings — Prep Time — Cook Time

Ingredients   Directions

NOTES

RECIPE:

Servings Prep Time Cook Time

Ingredients **Directions**

NOTES

RECIPE:

Servings   Prep Time   Cook Time

Ingredients   Directions

NOTES

RECIPE:

Servings | Prep Time | Cook Time

Ingredients | Directions

🗒 NOTES

RECIPE:

Servings　　　　　　　　Prep Time　　　　　　　　Cook Time

Ingredients　　Directions

NOTES

RECIPE:

Servings Prep Time Cook Time

Ingredients Directions

NOTES

RECIPE:

Servings | Prep Time | Cook Time

Ingredients | **Directions**

NOTES

RECIPE:

Servings　　　　　　Prep Time　　　　　　Cook Time

Ingredients　　Directions

NOTES

RECIPE:

Servings　　　　　　　　Prep Time　　　　　　　　Cook Time

Ingredients　　Directions

NOTES

RECIPE:

Servings | Prep Time | Cook Time

Ingredients

Directions

NOTES

RECIPE:

Servings | Prep Time | Cook Time

Ingredients | Directions

NOTES

RECIPE:

Servings | Prep Time | Cook Time

Ingredients

Directions

NOTES

RECIPE:

Servings   Prep Time   Cook Time

Ingredients   Directions

NOTES

RECIPE:

Servings Prep Time Cook Time

Ingredients Directions

NOTES

RECIPE:

Servings   Prep Time   Cook Time

Ingredients   Directions

NOTES

RECIPE:

Servings　　　　　　　Prep Time　　　　　　　Cook Time

Ingredients　　Directions

NOTES

RECIPE:

Servings | Prep Time | Cook Time

Ingredients | Directions

NOTES

RECIPE:

Servings　　　　　　　Prep Time　　　　　　　Cook Time

Ingredients　　Directions

NOTES

RECIPE:

Servings | Prep Time | Cook Time

Ingredients | **Directions**

NOTES

RECIPE:

Servings | Prep Time | Cook Time

Ingredients | Directions

NOTES

RECIPE:

Servings | Prep Time | Cook Time

Ingredients | Directions

NOTES

RECIPE:

Servings Prep Time Cook Time

Ingredients Directions

NOTES

RECIPE:

Servings　　　　　　　　　Prep Time　　　　　　　　　Cook Time

Ingredients　　Directions

NOTES

RECIPE:

Servings Prep Time Cook Time

Ingredients Directions

NOTES

RECIPE:

Servings   Prep Time   Cook Time

Ingredients

Directions

NOTES

RECIPE:

Servings　　　　　　　Prep Time　　　　　　　Cook Time

Ingredients　　Directions

NOTES

RECIPE:

Servings   Prep Time   Cook Time

Ingredients   Directions

NOTES

RECIPE:

Servings　　　　　Prep Time　　　　　Cook Time

Ingredients　　Directions

NOTES

RECIPE:

Servings   Prep Time   Cook Time

Ingredients   Directions

NOTES

RECIPE:

Servings Prep Time Cook Time

Ingredients Directions

NOTES

RECIPE:

Servings | Prep Time | Cook Time

Ingredients

Directions

NOTES

RECIPE:

Servings   Prep Time   Cook Time

Ingredients   **Directions**

NOTES

RECIPE:

Servings | Prep Time | Cook Time

Ingredients | Directions

NOTES

RECIPE:

Servings   Prep Time   Cook Time

Ingredients   Directions

NOTES

RECIPE:

Servings   Prep Time   Cook Time

Ingredients   Directions

NOTES

RECIPE:

Servings   Prep Time   Cook Time

Ingredients   Directions

NOTES

RECIPE:

Servings   Prep Time   Cook Time

Ingredients   **Directions**

NOTES

RECIPE:

Servings | Prep Time | Cook Time

Ingredients | Directions

NOTES

RECIPE:

Servings	Prep Time	Cook Time

Ingredients	**Directions**

NOTES

RECIPE:

Servings　　　　　　　　　Prep Time　　　　　　　　　Cook Time

Ingredients　　Directions

NOTES

RECIPE:

Servings   Prep Time   Cook Time

Ingredients

Directions

NOTES

RECIPE:

Servings Prep Time Cook Time

Ingredients **Directions**

NOTES

RECIPE:

Servings | Prep Time | Cook Time

Ingredients | Directions

NOTES

RECIPE:

Servings · Prep Time · Cook Time

Ingredients

Directions

NOTES

RECIPE:

Servings   Prep Time   Cook Time

Ingredients   Directions

NOTES

RECIPE:

Servings　　　　　　　　Prep Time　　　　　　　　Cook Time

Ingredients　　Directions

NOTES

RECIPE:

Servings · Prep Time · Cook Time

Ingredients

Directions

NOTES

RECIPE:

Servings | Prep Time | Cook Time

Ingredients | Directions

NOTES

RECIPE:

Servings | Prep Time | Cook Time

Ingredients | Directions

NOTES

RECIPE:

Servings | Prep Time | Cook Time

Ingredients | Directions

NOTES

RECIPE:

Servings　　　　　　　Prep Time　　　　　　　Cook Time

Ingredients　　　Directions

NOTES

RECIPE:

Servings　　　　　　　　Prep Time　　　　　　　　Cook Time

Ingredients　　Directions

NOTES

RECIPE:

Servings   Prep Time   Cook Time

Ingredients   **Directions**

NOTES

RECIPE:

Servings / Prep Time / Cook Time

Ingredients

Directions

NOTES

RECIPE:

Servings   Prep Time   Cook Time

Ingredients   Directions

NOTES

RECIPE:

Servings | Prep Time | Cook Time

Ingredients

Directions

NOTES

RECIPE:

Servings Prep Time Cook Time

Ingredients Directions

NOTES

RECIPE:

Servings	Prep Time	Cook Time

Ingredients

Directions

NOTES

RECIPE:

Servings Prep Time Cook Time

Ingredients Directions

NOTES

RECIPE:

Servings — Prep Time — Cook Time

Ingredients

Directions

NOTES

RECIPE:

Servings   Prep Time   Cook Time

Ingredients   Directions

NOTES

RECIPE:

Servings — Prep Time — Cook Time

Ingredients | Directions

NOTES

RECIPE:

Servings | Prep Time | Cook Time

Ingredients

Directions

NOTES

RECIPE:

Servings   Prep Time   Cook Time

Ingredients   **Directions**

NOTES

RECIPE:

Servings　　　　　Prep Time　　　　　Cook Time

Ingredients　　Directions

NOTES

RECIPE:

Servings Prep Time Cook Time

Ingredients Directions

NOTES

RECIPE:

Servings · Prep Time · Cook Time

Ingredients

Directions

NOTES

RECIPE:

Servings Prep Time Cook Time

Ingredients **Directions**

NOTES

RECIPE:

Servings | Prep Time | Cook Time

Ingredients

Directions

NOTES

RECIPE:

Servings　　　　　Prep Time　　　　　Cook Time

Ingredients　　Directions

NOTES

RECIPE:

Servings　　　　Prep Time　　　　Cook Time

Ingredients　　Directions

NOTES

RECIPE:

Servings Prep Time Cook Time

Ingredients Directions

NOTES

RECIPE:

Servings Prep Time Cook Time

Ingredients Directions

NOTES

RECIPE:

Servings　　　　　　　　Prep Time　　　　　　　　Cook Time

Ingredients　　Directions

NOTES

RECIPE:

Servings | Prep Time | Cook Time

Ingredients

Directions

NOTES

RECIPE:

Servings　　　　　Prep Time　　　　　Cook Time

Ingredients　　Directions

NOTES

RECIPE:

Servings Prep Time Cook Time

Ingredients Directions

NOTES

RECIPE:

Servings   Prep Time   Cook Time

Ingredients

Directions

NOTES

RECIPE:

Servings | Prep Time | Cook Time

Ingredients

Directions

NOTES

RECIPE:

Servings　　　　　　　Prep Time　　　　　　　Cook Time

Ingredients　　Directions

NOTES

RECIPE:

Servings | Prep Time | Cook Time

Ingredients

Directions

NOTES

RECIPE:

Servings | Prep Time | Cook Time

Ingredients

Directions

NOTES

RECIPE:

Servings   Prep Time   Cook Time

Ingredients   Directions

NOTES

RECIPE:

Servings | Prep Time | Cook Time

Ingredients

Directions

NOTES

RECIPE:

Servings   Prep Time   Cook Time

Ingredients

Directions

NOTES

RECIPE:

Servings — Prep Time — Cook Time

Ingredients

Directions

NOTES

RECIPE:

....

Servings · Prep Time · Cook Time

Ingredients · Directions

NOTES

RECIPE:

Servings | Prep Time | Cook Time

Ingredients

Directions

NOTES

RECIPE:

Servings   Prep Time   Cook Time

Ingredients   Directions

NOTES

RECIPE:

Servings　　　　　Prep Time　　　　　Cook Time

Ingredients　　Directions

NOTES

RECIPE:

Servings | Prep Time | Cook Time

Ingredients | Directions

NOTES

RECIPE:

Servings Prep Time Cook Time

Ingredients

Directions

NOTES

RECIPE:

Servings Prep Time Cook Time

Ingredients **Directions**

NOTES

RECIPE:

Servings Prep Time Cook Time

Ingredients Directions

NOTES

RECIPE:

Servings | Prep Time | Cook Time

Ingredients

Directions

NOTES

RECIPE:

Servings　　　　　　　　Prep Time　　　　　　　　Cook Time

Ingredients　　Directions

🍳 NOTES

RECIPE:

Servings · Prep Time · Cook Time

Ingredients | Directions

NOTES

RECIPE:

Servings | Prep Time | Cook Time

Ingredients

Directions

NOTES

RECIPE:

Servings　　　　　　　　Prep Time　　　　　　　　Cook Time

Ingredients　　Directions

🍳 NOTES

RECIPE:

Servings | Prep Time | Cook Time

Ingredients

Directions

📖 NOTES

RECIPE:

Servings   Prep Time   Cook Time

Ingredients   Directions

NOTES

RECIPE:

Servings | Prep Time | Cook Time

Ingredients

Directions

NOTES

RECIPE:

Servings | Prep Time | Cook Time

Ingredients | Directions

NOTES

RECIPE:

Servings · Prep Time · Cook Time

Ingredients

Directions

NOTES

KITCHEN CONVERSIONS
A guide to help you in the kitchen

SPOONS & CUPS

tsp	tbsp	fl oz	cup	pint	quart	gallon
3	1	1/2	1/16	1/32	-	-
6	2	1	1/8	1/16	1/32	-
12	4	2	1/4	1/8	1/16	-
18	6	3	3/8	-	-	-
24	8	4	1/2	1/4	1/8	1/32
36	12	6	3/4	-	-	-
48	16	8	1	1/2	1/4	1/16
96	32	16	2	1	1/2	1/8
-	64	32	4	2	1	1/4
-	256	128	16	8	4	1

MILLILITERS
(ROUNDED TO THE CLOSEST EQUIVALENT)

tsp	mL
1/2	2.5
1	5

tbsp	mL
1	15

oz	mL
2	60
4	115
6	150
8	230
10	285
12	340

cup	mL
1/4	60
1/2	120
2/3	160
3/4	180
1	240

GRAMS
(ROUNDED TO THE CLOSEST EQUIVALENT)

oz	g	lb
2	58	-
4	114	-
6	170	-
8	226	1/2
12	340	-
16	454	1

KITCHEN CONVERSIONS
A guide to help you in the kitchen

temperature conversion

°F	°C	°F	°C
225 °F	110 °C	375 °F	190 °C
250 °F	130 °C	400 °F	200 °C
275 °F	140 °C	425 °F	220 °C
300 °F	150 °C	450 °F	230 °C
325 °F	165 °C	475 °F	245 °C
350 °F	177 °C	500 °F	260 °C

Slow Cooker Conversion

Conventional Recipe Time	Slow Cooker Time On Low	Slow Cooker Time On High
15 to 30 mins.	4 to 6 hours	2 to 3 hours
35 to 45 mins.	6 to 8 hours	3 to 4 hours
50 mins. to 3 hrs.	8 to 10 hours	4 to 6 hours

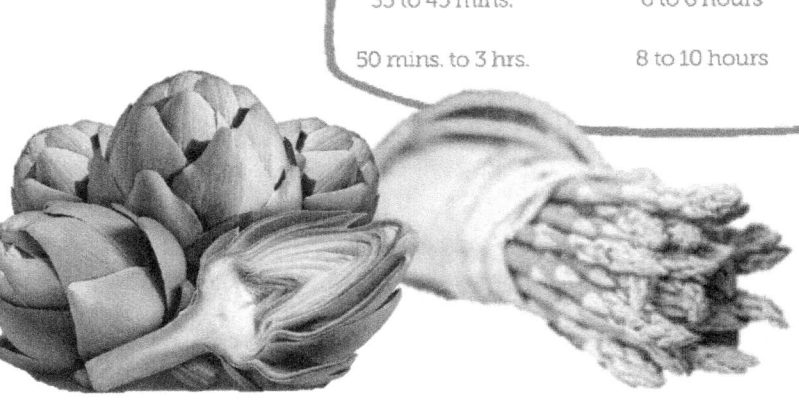
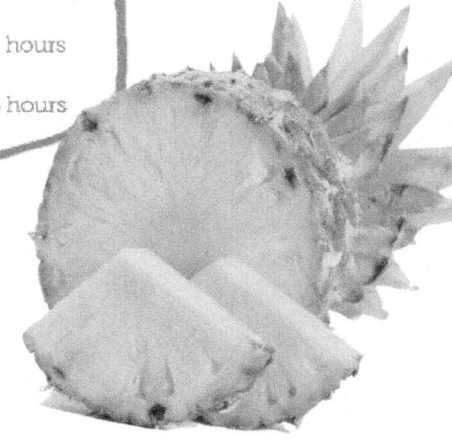

Copyright © 2019 Billionaire's Blank Cookbooks

Copyright © 2019 Motivational Affirmation Journals

All rights reserved.

No part of this publication may be reproduced, distributed or transmitted in any form or by any means, including photocopying, recording or other electronic or mechanical methods without prior written permission of the publisher. Except in the case of brief quotations embodied in critical reviews and certain other noncommercial uses permitted by copyright law.

- Printed in USA -

Made in the USA
Monee, IL
12 December 2019